A Hot New You!
In Only 12 Minutes a Day

An Easy Peasy Exercise Program for Women Over 40

By Ryder Management Inc.

Epigraph

"You only live once, but if you do it right, once is enough."
Mae West

"What the hell" is always the right answer?"
Marilyn Monroe

Table of Contents

Introduction

When we were young, muscle tone and the firmness that came with it, seemed to be more in reach than it is today. As we age and decide to be less active by not purposely exercising every day, our muscles become softer and more week and – horrors of horrors –flabby!

Did you know that a rounded and protruding abdomen is nothing more than weak stomach muscles allowing internal organs to sag forward?

Muscle condition is important to the way we look and feel and diet alone is not enough to alter sagging muscles and protruding abdomens. The best method of changing the way we look and feel is through a combination of both diet AND exercise.

Housework can involve a great deal of hard physical labor if you choose; however, it does not work all the muscles of the body. Some muscles get plenty of exercise while other muscles, such as the abdomen, get none.

With only 12 minutes a day, you can firm your muscles in your body, flatten your belly and become a Vibrant New You with energy and vitality.

This book consists of a progressive exercise program that requires performing the same series of 10 exercises within 12 minutes every day. The program includes 24 levels divided into Part A and Part B and is designed for ladies over 40.

Everyone is encouraged to begin at level 1 and once you master each level by allowing at least 7 – 14 days per level, you then proceed to the next level.

To assist you with staying committed to your daily 12 minute routine, this book includes a three step model that was developed by a much sought after business coach named Tom Bartow. The model is called **The Three Phases of Habit Formation** and will assist you with staying committed to your daily 12 minute routine and become a vibrant new you with energy and vitality.

Get Fit

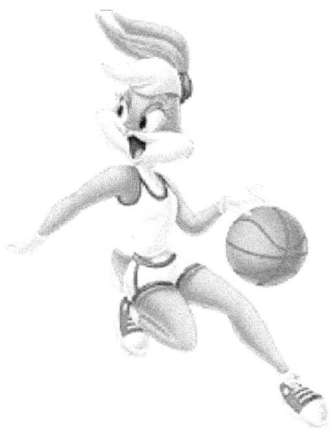

The following pages contain a description of ten exercises to complete within 12 minutes each day. The first chart includes the number of repetitions in each of levels 1 through 12. The program is designed to improve your general physical condition by increasing muscle tone, muscle strength, and muscle endurance. These exercises will also increase flexibility and the efficiency of your heart and reduce inches off your waist, hips and thighs.

Each exercise is included for its contribution to one or more of the following:

The first four exercises are for the purpose of improving and maintaining flexibility and mobility in specific areas of your body.

Exercise five is for strengthening your abs and for strengthening the front of your thigh muscles.

Exercise six strengthens your back, butt and the back

of your thighs.

Exercise seven focuses on both sides of your thighs. Both sides of your thigh muscles do not get enough of a work out in normal daily routines and in most sports.

Exercise eight focuses on your arms, shoulders and chest. This exercise also helps to strengthen your back and consequently, your abs.

Exercise nine focuses on your waist and hip muscles.

Exercise ten involves running and jumping and is primarily for conditioning your heart and lung muscles. This exercise also strengthens your leg muscles too.

The following page includes an exercise chart for the first 12 levels showing the number of repetitions required for each of the 10 exercises, in each level.

Everyone is encouraged to begin at level one. Please do not advance to the next level until you are able to **complete the existing level, without excessive strain or fatigue, within 12 minutes. It is recommended that you spend at least seven days on each level.**

If you feel sore or stiff, or become out of breathe at any time, slow down your progression.

Let's get started!

Part A – Your Exercise Program

Chart 1 – Levels 1 to 12

Level:	1	2	3	4	5	6	7	8	9	10
1	3	4	5	24	4	4	4	3	2	50
2	3	4	5	24	6	4	6	3	3	60
3	3	4	5	24	8	6	8	4	4	70
4	5	5	7	28	10	8	10	5	6	80
5	5	5	7	28	12	8	14	6	6	90
6	5	5	7	28	14	10	16	7	8	100
7	7	7	8	36	16	12	18	8	10	115
8	7	7	8	36	18	12	20	9	10	125
9	7	7	8	36	20	14	24	10	11	140
10	9	8	10	40	22	16	24	12	12	150
11	9	8	10	40	24	18	28	13	14	160
12	9	8	10	40	26	20	30	14	14	170
# Minutes per exercise	2	min		2	1	1	2	1	3	

The numbers 1-10 across the top on the above table refers to each of the ten exercises that are further explained on the pages that follow.

The numbers 1 -12 along the left hand side on the above table refers to the level number. You are encouraged to begin at level 1. The numbers in each box represents the number of repetitions, in each level, for each exercise. For example, exercise 1, Level 1, requires 3 repetitions and

Exercise 1, Level 12, requires 9 repetitions. More information on Exercise 1 follows this preamble.

Exercises 1 to 4 are warm-up exercises and all four exercises should be completed within two minutes or 30 seconds for each exercise. The total time required to complete all 10 exercises should be within a total of 12 minutes. The minimum number of days to spend on each level is one week.

Do not move to the next level until you are able to complete the prior level, without excessive strain or fatigue and within 12 minutes for a minimum of seven days before advancing.

Note that the number of minutes required to complete each exercise is indicated at the bottom of the above chart. Until you are able to complete each of the exercises within the stipulated time frame, without excessive stress or sweat, you are encouraged to remain in that particular level. The idea is to enjoy working out!

Included after exercise 10, is a blank table entitled "My Progress" for you to record your progress as you advance to Part B. Charting your progress is for the purpose of reminding you where you have left off plus to encourage you to use this routine on a regular daily basis for a more fit, toned beautiful YOU.

Exercise 1 – Toe Touching

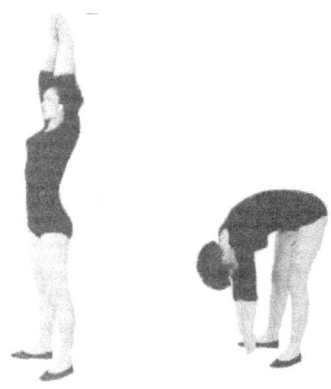

Exercise 1 – Toe Touching

Start: Stand tall with your feet approximately 12 inches apart, arms stretched up high above your head. Take a deep breath and bend forward to touch the ground between your feet, exhaling while doing so. Do not try to keep your knees straight, if it is a problem at first.

Return to starting position by inhaling and taking a deep breath, arms stretched high above your head.

How to Count: Each time you return to the starting position counts as one.

Level one requires three repetitions to be completed within thirty (30) seconds.

Exercise 2 – Knee Raising

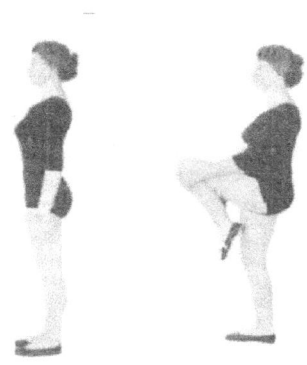

Exercise 2 – Knee Raises

Start: Stand tall with your hands at your sides and with feet together. Raise your left knee as high as possible, grasping your knee and shin with both hands. Pull leg toward your body. Make you that you keep your back straight throughout. Lower your left foot to the floor. Repeat with right leg. Continue this exercise by alternating legs; left then right.

Count: Raising both left and right knee counts as one. In other words, lifting your left and right leg counts as one repetition.

Level one requires five repetitions.

Exercise 3 – Side Bends

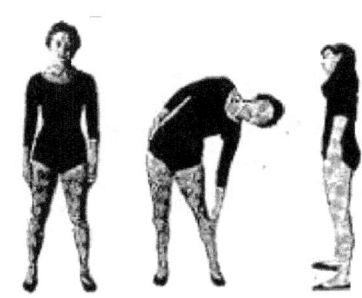

Exercise 3 – Side Bends

Start: Stand stall, feet 12 inches apart, hands at sides. Keeping your back straight and bend sideways from your waist to the **left** and slide your left hand down your left leg as far as you can. Return to starting position while inhaling until standing tall.

Slowly exhale as you bend down sideways on your **right** side, sliding your hand down your right leg as far as you can.

Continue by alternating left and then right.

Count: Bending to the left and then right counts as one.

Level one requires four repetitions (4 per side).

Level 12 requires ten repetitions (10 per side).

Exercise 4 – Arm Circles

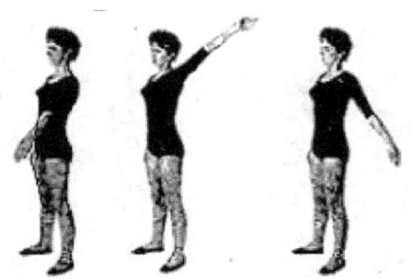

Exercise 4 – Arm Circles

Start: Stand stall; hands at your sides and your feet 12 inches apart. Make a large circle with your left arm. Do one quarter of the total required count with forward circles, and one quarter with backward circles. Repeat with your right arm.

Count: One full arm circle counts as one.

Level one requires 24 circles in total; 12 with each arm (and each arm is to do six forward and six backwards)

Level 12 requires 40 circles in total, 20 with each arm (and each arm is to do 10 forward and ten backwards)...

Exercise 5 – Partial Sit-ups

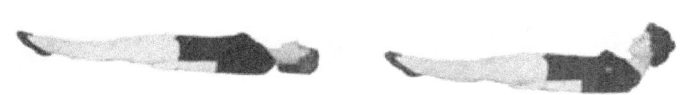

Exercise 5 – Partial Sit-ups

Start: Lie down on your back, legs straight and together with your arms at your side and take a deep breath.

Exhale as you raise your head, shoulders and feet up until you can see the heels of your feet. Lower your head and feet to the floor as you inhale, to begin again ….

Count: Each sit-up counts as one.

Level one requires four repetitions.

Level 12 requires 26 repetitions.

This exercise is for strengthening your abs and the front of your thighs.

Exercise 6 – Chest and Leg Raise

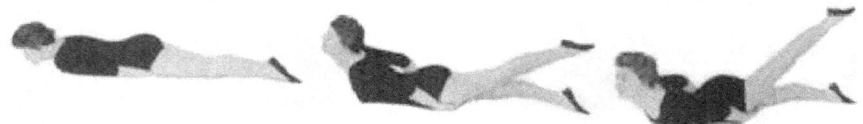

Exercise 6 – Chest and Leg Raise

Start: Lie face down, arms at your side with your hands under your thighs and your palms pressing against your thighs. Raise your head, shoulders and **left** leg as high as possible off the floor, keeping your leg straight. Lower it to the floor. Repeat raising your head, shoulders and **right** leg as high as possible. Continue by alternating each leg, left, then right.

Count: Each chest and leg raise, counts as one. Level one requires four repetitions.

This exercise will strengthens your back, butt and the back of your thighs

.

Exercise 7 – Side Leg Raise

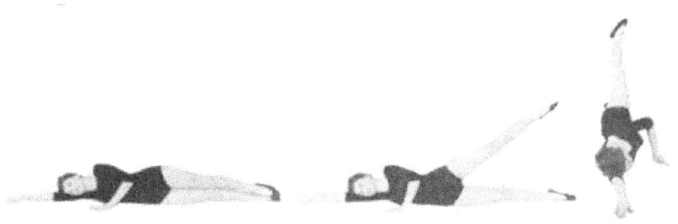

Exercise 7 – Side Leg Raise

Start: Lie on side, legs straight and together and your lower arm stretched above your head along the floor, using your top arm for balance. Raise your upper leg 18 – 24 inches and then lower it back to the starting position.

Count: Each leg raise counts as one. Do half the number of counts raising left leg. Roll over to your other side and do the other half number of counts raising your right leg. Level one requires a total of four repetitions.

Level 1 requires 4 repetitions

Level 12 requires 30 repetitions.

This exercise focuses on both sides of your thighs. Both sides of your thigh muscles do not get enough of a work out in normal daily routines and in most sports.

.

Exercise 8 – Push-ups

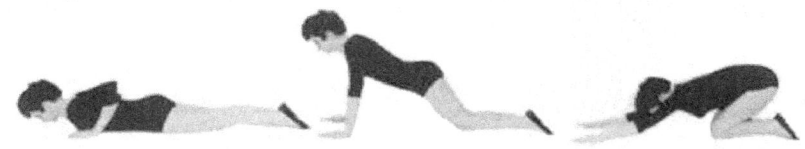

Exercise 8 – Push-ups

Start: Lie on floor, face down, legs straight and together, hands directly under your shoulders. Push your body up off the floor, until your arms are straight and then push back and sit on your heels, lowering your body to the floor. Return to starting position.

Count: Each return to the starting position counts as one repetition.

Level one requires a total of three repetitions.

Level 12 requires a total of 14 repetitions.

This exercise focuses on your arms, shoulders and chest. This exercise also helps to strengthen your back and consequently, your abs.

Exercise 9 – Leg Lifts

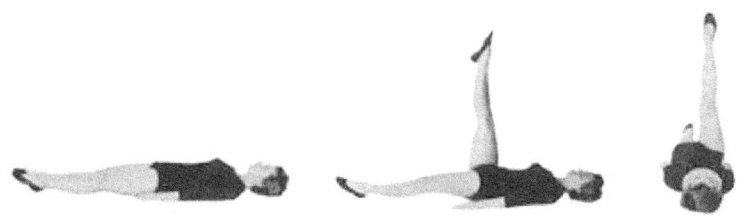

Exercise 9 – Leg Lifts

Start: Lie on your back, legs together and straight, toes pointed, arms at your side with your palms faced down. Raise your left leg until it is perpendicular to the floor, or as close as you can. Lower your left leg back down to the floor and repeat using your right leg. Continue alternating between your left legs, followed by your right leg.

Count: After raising your left leg and then your right counts as one repetition.

Level one requires two repetitions.

Level 12 requires 14 repetitions.

This exercise focuses on your waist and hip muscles.

Exercise 10 – Run and Hop

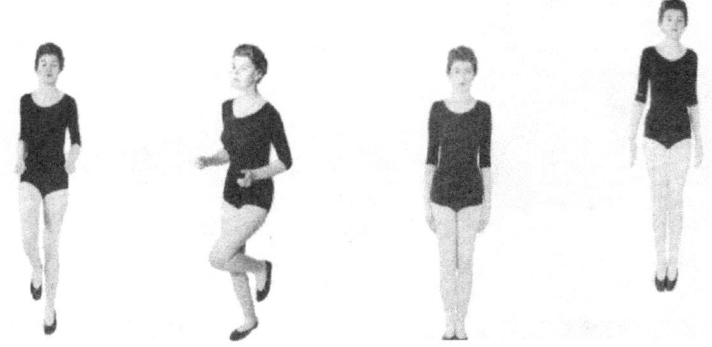

Exercise 10 – Run and Hop

Start: Stand tall with your feet together with your arms at your side. Starting with your left leg, run in one spot raising your feet at least six inches from the floor. (When running in one place, lift your knees forward, but don't just kick your heels backwards.)

Count: Each time your left foot touches the floor counts as one repetition.

Level one requires 50 repetitions. After each count of 50, do ten hops.

Level 12 requires 170 repetitions with 10 hops after each count of 50.

Hops: Hopping is done with both feet leaving the floor together. Try to hop at least four inches off the floor with each hop.

Note: In all running in one spot exercises, only the running steps count towards the indicated repetitions. Hopping is a bonus for your butt.

This exercise is primarily for conditioning your heart and lung muscles. This exercise also strengthens your leg muscles too.

My Progress – Chart 1

Level	Start date	Finish date	Comments
1			
2			
3			
4			
5			

6			
7			
8			
9			
10			
11			
12			

In addition to recording and keeping track of your progression through each of the 12 levels above, also record the following:

	Date	Height	Weight	Waist	Hips	Bust
Start						
Midway						
Finish						

Part B – Intermediate Level

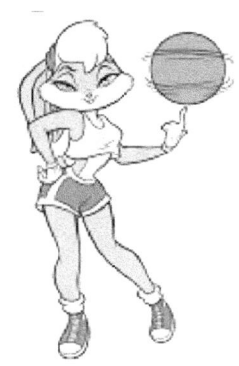

Part B, The Intermediate Level, includes the same basic ten exercises you performed previously in Part A, but they are at a more advanced level. The Intermediate Level includes levels 13 to 24 and is based on Chart 2 which follows.

Exercise one to four in Chart 2 comprises the warm-up exercises and should be completed within a total of two minutes or a total of 30 seconds each.

Exercises 5 through10 should be completed within a total of 10 minutes. This is your goal to strive for while in each level. You should not advance to the next level until you are able to complete the current level within 12 minutes, while still quite comfortable, ready for more.

Again, as in Part A, please do not move to the next level until you are able to complete your existing level without excessive strain, fatigue and , for Part B at least 14-28 days have been allowed for each level in Part B.

Remember that it is about the journey, not the destination that counts and it is important to make your journey enjoyable.

Chart 2 – Levels 13 to 24

Exercise number

Level	1	2	3	4	5	6	7	8	9	10
13	10	10	7	18	9	12	28	8	8	120
14	10	10	7	18	11	15	30	10	8	120
15	10	10	7	18	14	18	32	12	10	130
16	12	12	9	20	16	21	34	14	10	140
17	12	12	9	20	19	24	36	16	12	150
18	12	12	9	20	22	27	38	18	14	150
19	13	14	11	26	24	29	40	20	14	160
20	13	14	11	26	27	31	42	21	16	175
21	13	14	11	26	29	32	44	23	16	190
22	15	16	12	30	31	34	46	24	18	200
23	15	16	12	30	33	36	48	26	18	200
24	15	16	12	30	35	38	50	28	20	210
# Min Per Ex	2	Min	total		2	1	1	2	1	3

In order to ensure you are able to navigate through Chart 2, Levels 13 to 24, the following examples are provided

Level 13, Exercise 7 requires 28 repetitions whereas Level 22, Exercise 7 requires 46 requires 46 repetitions.

Please do not advance to the next level until you are able to complete your existing level with ease.

Exercise 1 – Intermediate Toe Touching

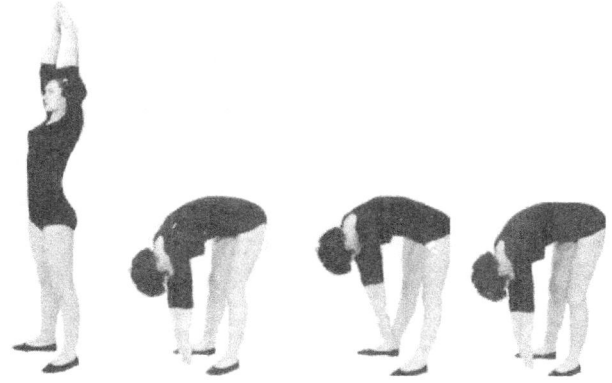

Chart 2 Exercise 1 – Intermediate Toe Touch

Start: Stand tall with your feet approximately 12 inches apart, arms stretched up high above your head. Take a deep breath and exhale while bending forward to touch the ground between your feet. Do not try to keep your knees straight, if it is a problem at first.

Return to starting position while inhaling and taking a deep breath, arms stretched high above your head.

Count: Each return to starting position counts as one.

Level 13 requires 10 repetitions in 30 seconds.

Level 24 requires 15 repetitions in 30 seconds.

Exercise 2 – Knee Raises

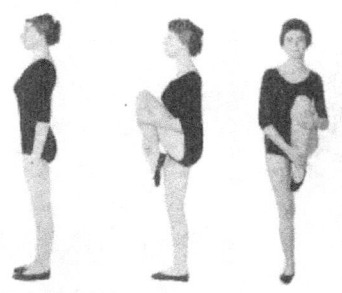

Chart 2 Exercise 2 Knee Raises

Start: Stand tall with your hands at your sides and with your feet together. Raise your left knee as high as possible, grasping knee and shin with both hands. Pull leg toward your body. Keep your back straight throughout. Lower your left foot to the floor. Repeat with your right leg. Continue by alternating legs; left then right.

Count: Raising both left and right knee counts as one.

Level 13 requires 10 repetitions in 30 seconds.

Level 24 requires 16 repetitions in 30 seconds.

Exercise 3 – Intermediate Side Bends

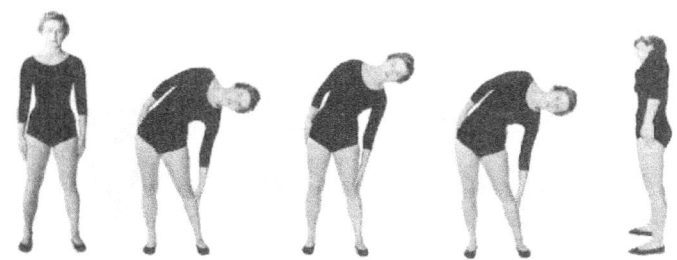

Chart 2 Exercise 3 Intermediate Side Bends

Start: Stand tall with your feet 12 inches apart, hands at sides. Keeping your back straight, bend sideways from your waist to the left and slide your left hand down your leg as far as possible. Bob up a few inches and press sideways and down again

Return to starting position and then bend downwards on your right side, sliding your hand down your leg as far as you can. Continue by alternating left and then right.

Count: Bending to the left and then right counts as one.

Level 13 requires 7 repetitions in 30 seconds.

Level 24 requires 12 repetitions in 30 seconds.

Exercise 4 – Arm Circles

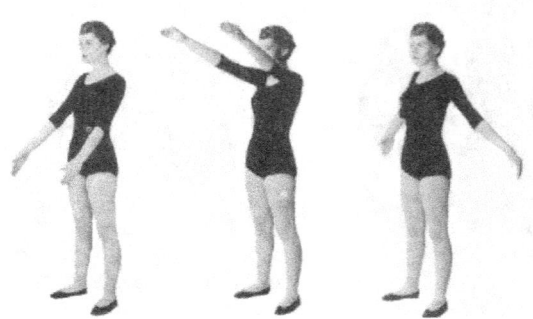

Chart 2 Exercise 4 Arm Circles

Start: Stand tall with your hands at sides and with feet 12 inches apart. Make a large circle with both arms at the same time, backwards and around. Do half the number of repetitions making backward circles and half making forward circles.

Count: Each full arm circle counts as one.

Level 13 requires 18 repetitions in 30 seconds.

Exercise 5 – Rocking Sit-ups

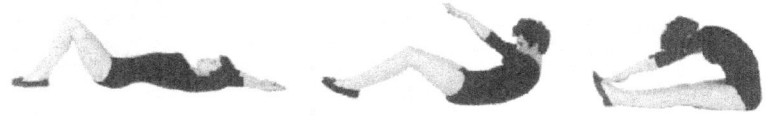

Chart 2 Exercise 5 Rocking Sit-ups

Start: Lie down on your back, legs straight and together with your arms at your side. Keeping your back as straight as possible move to a sitting position. Slide hands along legs during this movement finally reaching forward to try to touch toes with fingers. Return to starting position.

Count: Each return to starting position counts as one.

Level 13 requires 9 repetitions in two minutes.

Level 24 requires 35 repetitions.

This exercise is for strengthening your abs and the front of your thighs.

Exercise 6 – Chest and Leg Raises

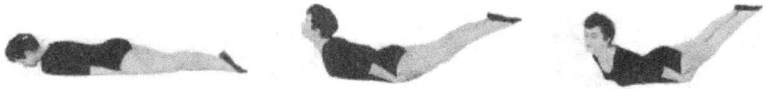

Chart 2 Exercise 6 Chest and Leg Raise

Start: Lie face down, arms at your sides under your thighs and with your palms pressing against your thighs. Raise your head, shoulders and both legs as high as you can off the floor, keeping your legs straight. Lower your legs and head to the floor and return to starting position. Repeat.

Count: Each return to the starting position counts as one repetition.

Level 13 requires 12 repetitions within 1 minute.

Level 24 requires 38 repetitions.

This exercise will strengthens your back, butt and the back of your thighs

Exercise 7 – Side Leg Raises

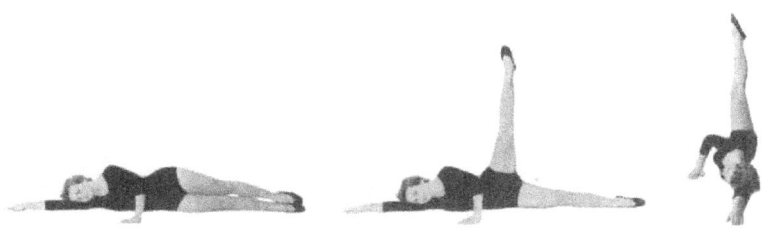

Chart 2 Exercise 7 Side Leg Raise

Start: Lie on side, legs straight and together and your lower arm stretched above your head along the floor, using your top arm for balance. Raise your upper leg until it is perpendicular to the floor or as close to that position as possible. Lower to starting position.

Count: Each leg raise counts as one. Do half the number of counts raising left leg. Roll over to your other side and do the other half number of counts raising your right leg.

Level 13 requires a total of 28 repetitions in 1 minute.

Level 24 requires a total of 50 repetitions.

This exercise focuses on both sides of your thighs. Both sides of your thigh muscles do not get enough of a work out in normal daily routines or in most sports.

Exercise 8 – Knee Push-ups

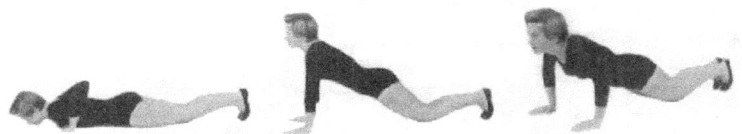

Chart 2 Exercise 8 Knee Push-ups

Start: Lie on floor, face down, legs straight and together, hands directly under your shoulders. Push your body up off the floor, until your arms are straightened. Keep hands and knees in contact with floor. . Return to starting position.

Count: Each return to the starting position counts as one repetition.

Level 13 requires a total of 8 repetitions in two minutes.

Level 24 requires a total of 28 repetitions

This exercise focuses on your arms, shoulders and chest. This exercise also helps to strengthen your back and consequently, your abs.

Exercise 9 – Leg Up and Over

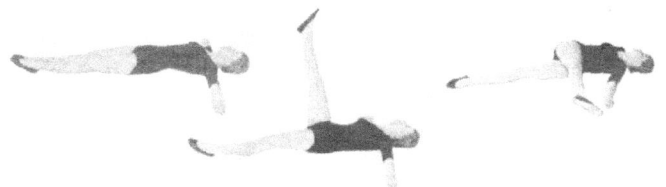

Chart 2 Exercise 9 Leg Up and Over

Start: Lie on your back, legs together and straight, toes pointed, arms stretched out sideways at shoulder level.

Lift your left leg high to a perpendicular position. Drop your raised leg over across your body and try to touch right hand with toes. Raise that leg back to a perpendicular position before returning it to the starting position. Repeat same movement with your right leg. Keep body and legs straight throughout, and shoulders on floor.

Count: Each return to starting position counts as one.

Level 13 requires 8 repetitions within one minute.

Level 24 requires 20 repetitions.

This exercise focuses on your waist and hip muscles.

Exercise 10 - Run and Stride Jumps

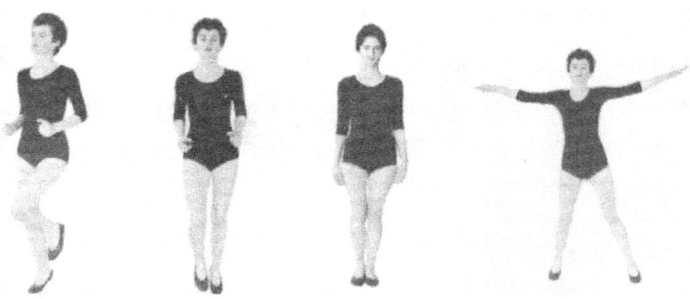

Chart 2 Exercise 10 Run and Stride Jumps

Start: Stand tall with your feet together with your arms at your side. Starting with your left leg, run in place raising your feet at least six inches from the floor. (When running in one place, lift your knees forward, but don't just kick your heels backwards.)

Count: Each time your left foot touches the floor counts as one repetition.

Level 13 requires 120 repetitions in 3 minutes. After each count of 50, do ten stride jumps.

Level 24 requires 210 repetitions with ten side jumps after each count of 50.

Stride jumps: Stride jump starts with feet together, arms at sides. Jump so that feet are about 18 inches apart when you land. At the same time as you jump, raise arms sideways to shoulder height. Jump again so that feet are together and arms are at sides when you land.

This exercise is primarily for conditioning your heart and lung muscles. This exercise also strengthens your leg muscles too.

My Progress – Chart 2

Level	Start date	Finish date	Comments
13			
14			
15			
16			
17			
18			
19			
20			
21			
22			
23			
24			

In addition to recording your progression through each of the 12 levels, also record the following, in order to record your progress throughout this program:

	Date	Height	Weight	Waist	Hips	Bust
Start						
Midway						
Finish						

Three Phases of Habit Formation

You are encouraged to perform each of the ten exercises in 12 minutes, every day. The benefits of looking and feeling great will be felt in no time. More importantly, your health will improve and your energy and vitality will return or increase.

To assist you with making the 12 minutes part of your lifestyle, consider the **three phases of habit formation**, a model developed by Tom Bartow, a highly sought after business coach. His 3 phase model can be summarized as follows:

Phase 1: The Honeymoon: is the beginning of anything new that you are excited about starting. This phase is usually the result of something inspiring. For example you are visualizing a slimmer; more firm you, with an abundance of energy!

Phase 2: The Fight Thru: is when inspiration tends to fade. Old habits are lurking around the corner making you wrestle whether to go back to old habits. The key to moving onto the third phase of habit formation is to win two or three "fight thru's". This is critical and necessary.

The three phase model of habit formation includes the following additional techniques to assist you with **winning your first fight thru:**

Phase 2 – Winning Your First Fight Thru

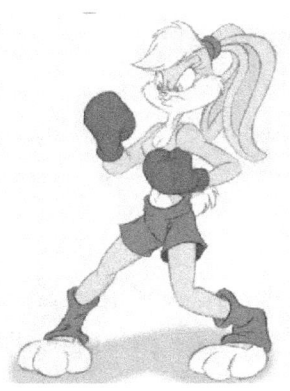

The key to advancing to the third and final stage using the Three Phase Model of Habit Formation, is winning two or more fight thru's. This is a very crucial step and the following three techniques are included to help you win:

Recognize: you are in a fight thru. Say out loud "I am in a fight thru and I will win this". Winning a fight thru will make it easier to win the next one. However, choosing to lose a fight thru sets you up to lose the next one.

Ask: yourself two questions: "How will I feel if I do this?" and "How will I feel if I don't do this?" Bring your emotions into this decision by letting yourself feel the positive in winning along with the negative in losing.

Big Picture: if the above two techniques have not propelled you back on track, think for a minute and imagine how your life will be in five years if you don't make any changes. Go into great detail and visualize it in your mind focusing on the worst case scenario.

Phase 3 – Second Nature

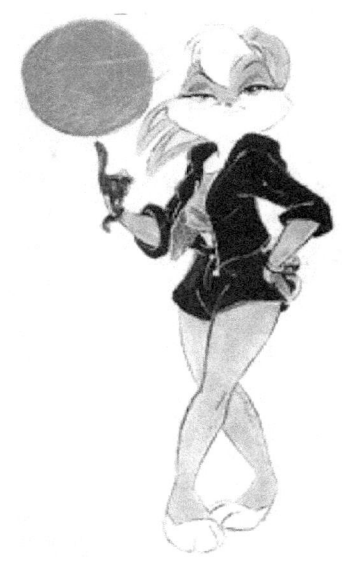

Phase 3 - Second Nature: occurs with feelings of being "in the groove", "on top of your game". Once in second nature however, it is important to be aware of three potential interruptions that can set you back to *fight thru*.

Three Potential Interruptions to your daily 12 minutes, include:

Discouragement: and allowing negative events be used as an excuse for skipping your daily 12 minute routine.

Disruptions: events such as vacations, holidays, weekends, illness or other changed patterns as a reason to skip your daily 12 minutes.

Too Cool For School: just because you achieved your goal and look hot and vibrant, is no reason to adopt the attitude that you are **too cool for school** and start skipping your daily 12 minutes.

If an interruption does set you back to fight thru, it may be necessary to win a few new fight thru's to help you comfortably move back to second nature.

Most people want positive habits to be as easy as brushing your teeth. Anything worth having is worth having to work for. As you advance through Chart 1, you will soon begin to feel and notice a change in you.

Conclusion

As you advance through each level in Part A, you should begin to consider adding a brisk 15 – 30 minute walk into your routine for increased and faster benefits. The most efficient way to accomplish this task is a quick, brisk walk through your neighborhood or around the block. Should it be cold outside, try using the fight thru technique to bundle up and walk a block or two before turning around to come home. If nothing else, it will leave you feeling invigorated.

Utilizing the program and techniques covered in this book, it is hoped that you will incorporate an exercise program, such as this one, into your daily life. In no time at all, you will begin to feel less fatigued and more vibrant. You will also be able to accomplish more tasks in a day with energy to spare; your leisure time will become more enjoyable; your posture will improve and you will begin to feel and look hot with a toned body that looks fabulous. These are just a few benefits.

By adjusting your diet to eliminate genetically modified food and toxic processed food, and commit to a 12 minute daily exercise routine, the beautiful new you will soon be staring you bake in the mirror. What are you waiting for? Why not start Exercise 1 right now?

Bonus

Working Out Versus Working in: The Importance of Both

By Talie Melnyk
www.TalieMelnyk.com

Let me introduce you to something that may change the way you approach exercise and bodywork. Let me introduce you to working out and working in. Believe it or not, they go hand in hand. They go together just like the two sides of the breath, the inhalation and the exhalation, the in and the out. Is one more important than the other? Can you have one without the other? For me, just like the breath, the answer is no. We are familiar with working out. It is part of our vernacular and hopefully for most of us, a regular part of our daily lives. But just as important is working in. We need to build both into our exercise routines, our bodywork, and into our habits. Google "working out," especially at this time of year, and there's a plethora of definitions, articles, tips, plans, routines, how to, how not to, etc. Now google "working in" and there's nothing there in terms of bodywork. It's likely because it's only a concept that we haven't embraced in the same way. We only focus on the external, the working out. And yet working out is only half of the work.

So let me define working in. Working in is the connection and exploration we make with the mind/breath/body and ultimately to the deeper part of ourselves. I'm not talking about the work one does with a therapist. However, regular working in will absolutely enhances one's mental and emotional health and well-being. Traditional mindful practices include yoga, Pilates, MELT, Feldenkrais and others along with a blend of any of these. One need not attend a Pilates or yoga class to make a connection to the mind/breath/body. It can happen within the structure of your regular workout. How? By connecting to and opening the expression of your breath, as well as focusing on the quality of each movement you make. Many just throw the sneakers on, the workout wear on, the headphones on, and disconnect to everything below the neck. We're taught that exercise is supposed to be really uncomfortable and, if you go along with some philosophies, painful. We've all heard the "no pain, no gain" approach. The goal is to just get through it whether it's the class, the workout, or the run. It's going to hurt and we want to feel as little as possible. Sound familiar?

Consider this: Instead of just throwing the sneakers and the headphones on and tuning out, try tuning in. Tune into your breath and the quality of each inhalation and exhalation. Tune into each rep, each step, each movement, and be present with each. When we are present and connected to our breath and our movement, change happens. We quiet the mind and all its chatter and are better able to replace negative self-talk with positive reinforcement. We quiet the nervous system and therefore the stress response in the body. We are able to challenge ourselves in the working out and better able to embrace the challenge when we are also working in. We begin to truly live in our bodies. Most importantly, we gain confidence in ourselves and make choices that are better for us, not just in the gym, but in all the other things we do.

Talie Melnyk is a certified movement specialist, residing in Brooklyn, NY. She assists women and special needs populations reach optimum health and mobility. Originally from Calgary, Alberta, Talie fell in love with the art of solo theatre after taking Gretchen's Cryer's "Writing for Solo Performance" and recently created, wrote and performed "Maison des Reves" in New York and Canada. www.taliemelnyk.com

The Food We Eat

White Sugar and Artificial Sweeteners

It should come as no surprise to learn that artificial sweetener marketers have been trying to persuade us into thinking that artificial sweeteners are a necessity for our individual weight control aspirations; however, they leave out the fact that their artificial sweeteners have the effect of harming our immune system and rob our bones of valuable minerals.

In 1957, Dr. William Coda Martin tried to answer the question: "When is a food a food and when is it a poison?"

Dr. Martin, in answering that question, responded as follows:

"Medically speaking, any substance applied to the body, ingested or developed within the body, which causes or may cause disease, is a poison." Dr. Martin went on to state in 1957, "Physically speaking, a poison is any substance which inhibits the activity of a catalyst which is a minor substance, chemical or enzyme that activates a reaction."

It should be noted that in 1957, Dr. Martin classified refined sugar as a poison since it is *"depleted of its life forces, vitamins and minerals, leaving an un-digestible refined carbohydrate."* He further stated: *"Refined sugar is lethal when ingested by humans because it provides only that which nutritionists describe as "empty" or "naked" calories. It lacks the natural minerals which are present in the sugar beet or cane. In addition, sugar is worse than nothing because it drains and leaches the body of precious vitamins and minerals through the demand its digestion, detoxification and elimination makes upon one's entire system."*

In view of the above, and in terms of Beautiful New YOU, it is strongly urged that you eliminate refined white sugar and artificial sweetener from your diet immediately. Consider including organic honey, coconut sugar, organic maple syrup or stevia as natural replacements since all these natural substitutes contain nutritional benefits required by our body and includes essential amino acids.

The Gluten and Muffin Belly Link

Despite what we have been led to believe, wheat is far from a health food item!

In fact, wheat and wheat products, such as most cereals, bread and any similar products, does NOT do your body good!!! Not anymore. Monsanto and wheat producers have changed wheat in dramatic ways. In the old days, wheat grew to at least four feet tall. Today, wheat rarely grows beyond two feet tall.

Dr. William Davis, a cardiologist or heart doctor, author and crusader of health, has stated:

"The food we eat is making us sick and the agencies that are providing us with the guidelines on what to eat are giving dangerous advice with devastating health consequences. YOU can change that

today. " http://beforeitsnews.com/health/2013/03/wheat-gmos-getting-us-all-sick-gluten-intolerance-2477592.html

GMO OMG

Despite being told our food products are not "genetically modified" (GM), "herbicide tolerant (HT)" crops were developed to survive applications of certain herbicides that previously would have destroyed the crop along with the unwanted weeds. Herbicide tolerant corn (a.k.a. genetically modified corn) has accelerated in use since 1996 and has reached 90 percent of US corn acreage in 2014."

In addition to herbicide tolerant crops, such as corn, "insect resistant crops containing the gene from the soil bacterium BT ((Bacillus thuringiensis) have been available for corn and cotton since 1996. These bacteria produce a protein that is toxic to specific insects, protecting the plant over its entire life. Plantings of Bt corn grew from about 8 percent of U.S. corn acreage in 1997 to 26 percent in 1999, then fell to 19 percent in 2000 and 2001, before climbing to 29 percent in 2003 and 90 percent in 2014."
http://www.ers.usda.gov/data-products/adoption-of-genetically-engineered-crops-in-the-us/recent-trends-in-ge-adoption.aspx

GM Corn is now prevalent in our everyday lives and on every supermarket shelf. GM corn includes almost every item of processed food due to GM corn syrup. GM corn is also fed to the livestock we buy including beef, pork and poultry.

Does GM food make us fat? According to the health authorities, genetically modified food has no effect on humans. That being said, according to Natural News:

"If you don't know you're not eating organic, GMO-free foods, then you likely consume them often and have been for years. Still, even if you've not yet manifested symptoms related to the many health complications associated with GMO consumption, your body is probably already under their influence. Foreign materials - in this case, "genetic foreign materials" - cause the immune system to work harder than usual to keep you from experiencing the inevitable consequences, which can be as serious as organ damage, diabetes, infertility, cancer and death. Studies so far suggest it's really only a matter of time before something goes terribly awry. Unfortunately, most corn, soy (as in the dairy-alternative milk, tofu, etc. much beloved by vegans), wheat and canola produced these days are genetically modified and it would probably be best to avoid them altogether. You'll know your foods are GMO-free if they bear either a label reading "100% organic" or the "Non-GMO Verified" logo."
http://www.naturalnews.com/038237_GMOs_making_yo u_fat_processed_foods.html#ixzz3Otg7FkK1

GMO Timeline

We have been falsely assured that our food has not been genetically modified. This brings to mind the following quotation:

"If you become aware of a lie and you do nothing to expose the lie, you then become part of that lie." Not me!

Although it was in 1935 when a Russian scientist - named Andrei Nikolaevitch Belozersky - isolated pure DNA, it wasn't until 1975 when guidelines for the safe use of GE DNA were established.

1980 – Due to a court case between a genetics engineer at General Electric and the U.S. Patent Office, the then pending patent was settled by a 5-to-4 Supreme Court ruling, allowing for the first patent on a living organism. The GMO in question was a bacterium with an appetite for crude oil, ready to gobble up spills.

1982 – FDA Approves First GMO -*Humulin*, insulin produced by genetically engineered E. coli bacteria. 1982 was the year it appeared, for the first time, on the market.

1994 – GMO Hits Grocery Stores

1996 – Introduction of GMO-Resistant Weeds

1999 – GMO Food Crops Dominate

2003 – GMO-Resistant Pests

2011 – BT Toxin in Humans

2012 – Farmer Wins Court Battle

2014 – GMO Patent Expires

Note!

According to Monsanto's website, their first generation "Roundup Ready soybeans, the world's most widely adopted biotech trait, planted by farmers on billions of acres since 1996—comes off patent in 2015."

ABOUT THE AUTHOR

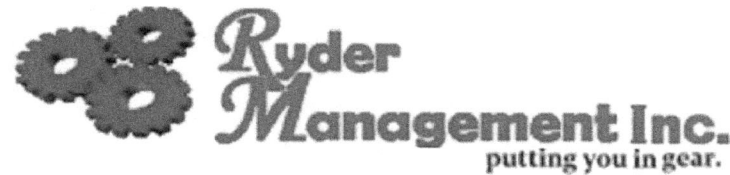

    Ryder Management Inc. (Rydermgt or RMI) is a Canadian Controlled Private Corporation (CCPC) based in London, ON Canada. As an "umbrella" organization, RMI brings together a group of authors whom are professionals in their respective fields and are writing with the primary goal of providing books that educate, comfort and offer assurance that natural health remedies do exist and are an effective and safe way to regain, obtain and maintain one's health.

    Other books written by RMI include *"Just Soup: Stocks, Broth and NutriBullet Blended Soups"*; *NutriBullet Recipes; Cinnamon for Health*, *"Recipes for Hemp Seeds: Recipes for the #1 Superfood on the Planet"*; among others. The total list of books can be found at Rydermgt's author page at Amazon's Author Central

www.amazon.com/author/rydermgt.

Or visit us at http://rydermanagement.ca

If you enjoyed this book, tell others! If not, tell us.